CHAIR PILATES FOR MEN OVER 50

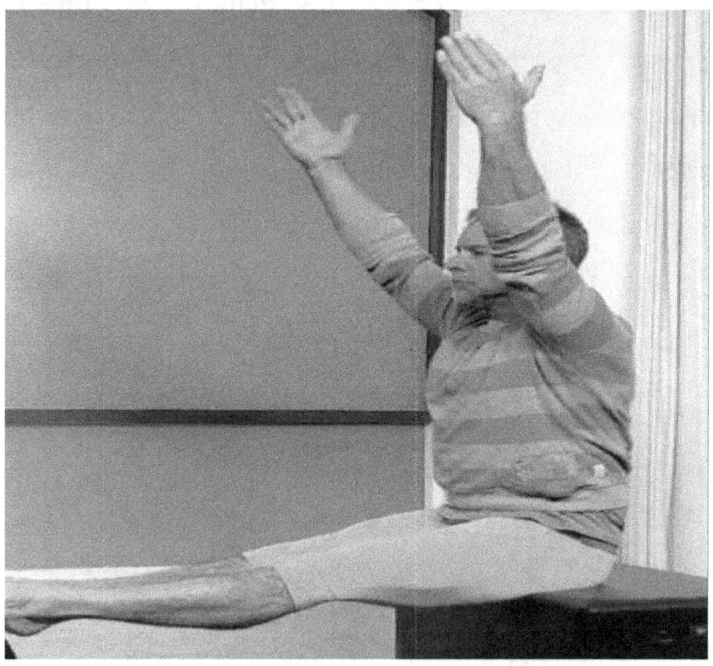

The Complete Guide For Beginners And Seniors To Build Strength, Enhance Flexibility And Increase Performance

Randy T. Lucas

Table of Contents

INTRODUCTION

Picture this: a man in his early 50s, once energetic and spry, now feeling the toll of a life filled with work, responsibilities, and perhaps a few too many rounds of golf on the weekends. His joints ache, and his back sometimes protests when he rises from his favorite armchair. Frustrated by the limitations he feels creeping in, he longs to regain his vitality and strength. Enter chair pilates.

In a world where fitness seems tailored for the young and athletic, chair pilates for men over 50 emerges as a beacon of hope. It's not just about the exercises; it's about rediscovering freedom in movement, reclaiming a zest for life, and embracing wellness in a way that respects the body's unique needs at this stage.

Imagine our man, hesitant at first, sitting on his comfortable armchair, skeptically eyeing the exercises outlined in this guide. As he starts incorporating these simple yet effective chair pilates routines into his daily routine, something miraculous happens. His body gradually remembers what it's like to move with ease. Those persistent joint pains start to diminish, his posture improves, and his energy levels soar. But it's not just the physical transformation. Chair pilates for men over 50 offers something deeper—a sense of rejuvenation that permeates his entire being. As he engages with each exercise, he rediscovers a connection between mind and body, feeling a renewed sense of confidence and inner balance. Suddenly, life feels vibrant again.

In this comprehensive guide, we'll explore how chair pilates specifically tailored for men over 50 can unlock a world of benefits which is increased flexibility, improved balance, enhanced core strength, and a newfound sense of vitality. We'll delve into exercises meticulously designed to cater to the unique requirements and challenges faced by men in this age group.

Whether you're a beginner or already familiar with pilates, this guide is a companion on your journey towards a healthier, more vibrant life. Join us as we delve into the transformative power of chair pilates, a gateway to a fitter body, a clearer mind, and a more fulfilling life, no matter the age.

CHAPTER 1

Understanding chair pilates

Chair pilates is a modified form of traditional pilates, tailored to accommodate individuals who may have limited mobility or prefer a seated workout. This gentle yet effective exercise regimen focuses on strengthening muscles, enhancing flexibility, and improving posture using a chair as the primary prop. It incorporates a series of controlled movements and breathing techniques, emphasizing the mind-body connection.

Understanding chair pilates involves recognizing its adaptability and versatility. It caters to various fitness levels, making it accessible for men over 50 seeking to improve their physical well-being. By engaging in seated exercises that target core strength, flexibility, and balance, participants can experience the benefits of pilates without the need for complex equipment or extensive floor exercises. Chair pilates offers a gateway to increased vitality, reduced stress, and better overall health, making it a welcoming and beneficial fitness option for those seeking a gentle yet impactful workout regimen.

Safety Tips and Precautions

1. Consult a healthcare professional: Before starting any exercise regimen, especially if you have underlying health conditions, it's essential to consult with your doctor or a healthcare professional. They can provide guidance specific to your health status and advise if chair pilates is suitable for you.

2. Start slowly: Begin with gentle exercises and gradually increase the intensity or duration as your body adjusts. Rushing into advanced movements can increase the risk of injury, particularly for those who have been inactive for some time.

3. Listen to your body: Pay attention to how your body feels during the exercises. If you experience pain, discomfort, or dizziness, stop immediately and reassess your form.

Discomfort during exercise is common, but sharp or shooting pain is not.

4. Maintain proper form: Focus on correct posture and technique during each movement. Proper alignment reduces strain on muscles and joints, minimizing the risk of injury. If unsure about the correct form, seek guidance from a certified instructor.

5. Use a sturdy chair: Ensure the chair you use is stable, sturdy, and without wheels. A solid, armless chair with a flat seat is ideal for chair pilates. Avoid using chairs that could tip or slide during exercises.

6. Wear appropriate clothing: Opt for comfortable, breathable clothing that allows for a full range of motion. Loose or baggy attire might get caught or hinder movement, while tight clothing may restrict blood flow.

7. Breathe mindfully: Focus on controlled breathing throughout the exercises. Proper breathing helps oxygenate muscles and aids in relaxation. Avoid holding your breath during movements, as it can increase blood pressure and tension.

8. Modify as needed: Adapt exercises to suit your individual needs and limitations. If a movement causes discomfort or is too challenging, modify it or seek alternatives that work for your body.

9. Stay hydrated: Drink water before, during, and after your chair pilates session to stay hydrated. Dehydration can lead to muscle cramps and fatigue.

10. Allow for rest and recovery: Give your body time to rest between sessions. Overexertion can lead to muscle strain or injury. Aim for a balanced routine that includes rest days to allow for recovery.

Benefits Of Chair Pilates For Men

1. Improved Flexibility: Chair pilates incorporates stretching and range-of-motion exercises that enhance flexibility, helping to counteract stiffness commonly experienced with age. This increased flexibility can improve posture and overall mobility.

2. Enhanced Core Strength: The core muscles play a crucial role in stability and balance. Chair pilates targets these muscles, leading to improved core strength. A stronger core can alleviate back pain and support better posture.

3. Better Balance and Stability: As men age, balance can become compromised. Chair pilates focuses on exercises that improve balance, reducing the risk of falls and enhancing overall stability, crucial for daily activities.

4. Gentle on Joints: Chair pilates offers a low-impact workout, making it gentler on the joints compared to other forms of exercise. This makes it suitable for individuals dealing with joint issues or arthritis.

5. Increased Muscle Strength: Regular practice of chair pilates helps in building and toning muscles without putting excessive strain on the body. Stronger muscles assist in supporting the body and performing daily tasks more efficiently.

6. Stress Reduction: Chair pilates emphasizes mindful movement and controlled breathing, promoting relaxation and reducing stress levels. This mind-body connection fosters a calmer state of mind and overall mental well-being.

7. Improved Posture: Poor posture is a common issue as people age. Chair pilates focuses on aligning the body correctly, strengthening muscles that support good posture. This leads to improved spinal alignment and decreased strain on the back.

8. Enhanced Mental Focus: Engaging in chair pilates requires concentration on movement and breathing, fostering mental focus and mindfulness. This mental clarity can improve cognitive function and overall mental sharpness.

9. Boosted Energy Levels: Regular practice of chair pilates can increase energy levels by promoting circulation and oxygen flow throughout the body. This revitalization is particularly beneficial for combating fatigue and maintaining vitality.

10. Customizable and Accessible: Chair pilates can be adapted to accommodate various fitness levels and physical abilities. Its accessibility makes it an ideal exercise regimen for men over 50, allowing for gradual progression and modification as needed.

WARM-UP EXERCISES

1. Shoulder Rolls

- Starting Position:

Sit comfortably in the chair with feet flat on the floor and hands resting on thighs.

- Steps:

Inhale, lift shoulders towards the ears, roll them back in a circular motion, and then down. Exhale as you complete the rotation.

- Repetition:

8-10 times clockwise, then 8-10 times counterclockwise.

- Purpose:

This exercise helps loosen tight shoulder muscles, improves flexibility, and reduces tension in the upper body.

2. Seated Torso Twist

- Starting Position:

Sit upright in the chair, feet planted firmly on the floor, and hands resting on the sides of the chair or across the chest.

- Steps:

Inhale, twist gently to the right from the waist, keeping the hips facing forward. Exhale and return to the center. Repeat on the other side.

- Repetition:

5-8 times on each side.

- Purpose:

It stretches the spine, increases spinal mobility, and helps warm up the back muscles.

3. Ankle Circles

- Starting Position:

Sit comfortably with feet flat on the floor.

- Steps:

Lift one foot and rotate the ankle in a circular motion, first clockwise and then counterclockwise. Repeat with the other foot.

- Repetition:

8-10 circles in each direction for each ankle.

- Purpose:

Ankle circles improve ankle flexibility, strengthen the lower leg muscles, and stimulate blood circulation in the feet and ankles.

4. Knee Lifts

- Starting Position:

Sit tall in the chair with feet flat on the floor.

- Steps:

Lift one knee towards the chest while keeping the back straight. Lower the foot back to the floor. Alternate between legs.

- Repetition:

8-10 lifts for each leg.

- Purpose:

This exercise warms up the hip flexors, activates the core muscles, and improves circulation in the lower body.

5. Deep Breathing

- Starting Position:
Sit comfortably, relax your shoulders, and rest your hands on your thighs.

- Steps:
Inhale deeply through the nose, expanding your belly, then exhale slowly through the mouth, contracting the abdominal muscles.

- Repetition:
5-8 deep breaths.

- Purpose:
Deep breathing oxygenates the body, relaxes the mind, and prepares for the workout by increasing oxygen flow to the muscles.

CHAPTER 2

CHAIR PILATES

1. Seated Marching

- Starting Position:
Sit tall in the chair, feet flat on the floor, and hands resting on thighs.

- Steps:
Lift one knee towards the chest, then lower it while lifting the other knee. Continue alternating legs in a marching motion.

- Repetition:
10-12 marches per leg (20-24 total).

- Purpose:
Strengthens the core muscles, improves hip flexor mobility, and increases circulation in the lower body.

2. Seated Leg Extensions

- Starting Position:

Sit on the edge of the chair with feet flat on the floor and hands resting on the sides of the chair for support.

- Steps:

Straighten one leg out in front of you, hold briefly, then return to the starting position. Alternate legs.

- Repetition:

8-10 extensions per leg.

- Purpose:

Targets the quadriceps and hamstrings, enhancing leg strength and stability.

3. Seated Side Bends

- Starting Position:

Sit upright in the chair, feet flat on the floor, and hands by your sides or lightly resting on the chair.

- Steps:

Inhale, reach one arm up and over towards the opposite side, bending sideways. Return to the center and alternate sides.

- Repetition:

6-8 bends on each side.

- Purpose:

Stretches the side torso muscles, improves spinal flexibility, and engages the obliques.

4. Seated Torso Circles

- Starting Position:

Sit comfortably with feet flat on the floor and hands resting on thighs.

- Steps:

Inhale as you lean forward, exhale as you circle to the right, lean back, circle to the left, and return to the starting position.

- Repetition:

5-6 circles in one direction, then reverse.

- Purpose:

Increases mobility in the spine, massages the abdominal organs, and strengthens the core muscles.

5. Seated Shoulder Squeezes

- Starting Position:

Sit tall in the chair with feet flat on the floor, hands resting on thighs, or holding onto the sides of the chair.

- Steps:

Inhale, squeeze the shoulder blades together, and gently push the chest forward. Exhale and release.

- Repetition:

10-12 squeezes.

- Purpose:

Relieves tension in the upper back, strengthens the muscles around the shoulder blades, and improves posture.

6. Seated Knee Lifts with Twist

- Starting Position:

Sit tall in the chair, feet flat on the floor, and hands behind your head or on the sides of the chair.

- Steps:

Lift one knee towards the chest while twisting your torso to touch the opposite elbow to the knee. Alternate between knees and elbows.

- Repetition:

8-10 lifts with twists on each side.

- Purpose:

Engages the abdominal muscles, improves core strength, and enhances rotational mobility in the torso.

7. Seated Chest Opener

- Starting Position:

Sit upright with feet flat on the floor and interlace fingers behind your back, gently straightening your arms.

- Steps:

Inhale, lift the chest and arms slightly, stretching the front of the chest. Exhale and release.

- Repetition:

Hold the stretch for 15-20 seconds, repeating 2-3 times.

- Purpose:

Stretches the chest muscles, counteracting the effects of hunching forward and promoting better posture.

8. Seated Heel Raises

- Starting Position:

Sit comfortably in the chair, feet flat on the floor.

- Steps:

Lift both heels off the ground, rising onto the balls of your feet. Lower them back down.

- Repetition:

12-15 heel raises.

- Purpose:

Strengthens the calf muscles, improves ankle stability, and enhances lower leg strength.

9. Seated Arm Circles

- Starting Position:

Sit tall with feet flat on the floor, arms extended out to the sides at shoulder height.

- Steps:

Make small circular motions with the arms, rotating them forward for several repetitions, then reverse the direction.

- Repetition:

8-10 circles in each direction.

- Purpose:

Warms up the shoulder joints, improves shoulder mobility, and engages the deltoid muscles.

10. Seated Pelvic Tilts

- Starting Position:

Sit on the edge of the chair, feet flat on the floor, and hands resting on thighs.

- Steps:

Inhale, tilt the pelvis forward, arching the lower back slightly. Exhale and tilt the pelvis backward, rounding the lower back. Alternate between the two movements.

- Repetition:

10-12 pelvic tilts.

- Purpose:

Mobilizes the spine, strengthens the core, and improves awareness of pelvic alignment.

11. Seated Arm Raises

- Starting Position:

Sit comfortably with feet flat on the floor and arms resting by your sides.

- Steps:

Inhale, raise both arms straight out to the sides or in front of you. Exhale and lower the arms back down.

- Repetition:

8-10 arm raises.

- Purpose:

Strengthens the shoulder muscles, improves shoulder mobility, and enhances posture.

12. Seated Abdominal Twists

- Starting Position:

Sit tall with feet flat on the floor, interlace fingers behind the head, and elbows out to the sides.

- Steps:

Inhale, rotate your torso to one side, bringing the opposite elbow towards the outside of the knee. Exhale and return to the center. Alternate sides.

- Repetition:

6-8 twists on each side.

- Purpose:

Engages the obliques, enhances core strength, and increases spinal mobility.

13. Seated Hip Flexor Stretch

- Starting Position:

Sit at the edge of the chair, with one foot planted on the floor and the other ankle resting on the opposite knee.

- Steps:

Lean forward slightly, keeping the back straight, and feel the stretch in the crossed leg's hip and buttock.

- Repetition:

Hold the stretch for 20-30 seconds per leg, repeating 2-3 times.

- Purpose:

Stretches and relaxes the hip flexor muscles, improving hip mobility and flexibility.

14. Seated Back Extension

- Starting Position:

Sit tall in the chair, hands behind your head or on your thighs.

- Steps:

Inhale, gently arch your back, lifting your chest and looking slightly upward. Exhale and return to the starting position.

- Repetition:

8-10 back extensions.

- Purpose:

Helps counteract sitting-related back stiffness, improves spinal mobility, and strengthens the back muscles.

15. Seated Wrist and Hand Stretches

- Starting Position:

Sit tall in the chair, palms facing up on your thighs or resting on the chair arms.

- Steps:

Gently stretch and flex your wrists and fingers, moving them in circles or stretching each finger individually.

- Repetition:

Perform 5-6 stretches for each hand.

- Purpose:

Alleviates tension in the hands and wrists, improves joint mobility, and helps prevent discomfort from repetitive movements.

16. Seated Oblique Crunches

- Starting Position:

Sit tall in the chair, feet flat on the floor, and hands lightly behind the ears.

- Steps:

Inhale, twist the torso to one side, bringing the elbow towards the hip. Exhale and return to the starting position. Alternate sides.

- Repetition:

8-10 crunches on each side.

- Purpose:

Targets the oblique muscles, strengthens the core, and improves lateral flexibility.

17. Seated Hip Circles

- Starting Position:

Sit comfortably with feet flat on the floor.

- Steps:

Slowly circle the hips in a clockwise direction, then reverse the movement to counterclockwise circles.

- Repetition:

6-8 circles in each direction.

- Purpose:

Increases mobility in the hip joints, improves hip flexibility, and loosens hip muscles.

18. Seated Calf Raises

- Starting Position:

Sit tall in the chair with feet flat on the floor.

- Steps:

Lift both heels off the ground, rising onto the balls of your feet. Lower them back down.

- Repetition:

12-15 calf raises.

- Purpose:

Strengthens the calf muscles, improves ankle stability, and promotes lower leg strength.

19. Seated Leg Crosses

- Starting Position:

Sit upright in the chair with feet flat on the floor.

- Steps:

Cross one leg over the other at the ankle or knee, feeling a gentle stretch in the hips. Switch legs after a few seconds.

- Repetition:

Hold each leg cross for 15-20 seconds, alternating sides.

- Purpose:

Stretches the hips and glutes, increases hip flexibility, and reduces tension in the lower body.

20. Seated Neck Stretch

- Starting Position:

Sit tall in the chair, shoulders relaxed and feet flat on the floor.

- Steps:

Tilt your head to one side, bringing your ear towards your shoulder, feeling a gentle stretch along the opposite side of the neck. Alternate sides.

- Repetition:

Hold each stretch for 15-20 seconds, repeating 2-3 times on each side.

- Purpose:

Relieves tension in the neck muscles, improves neck flexibility, and helps alleviate stiffness.

21. Seated Side Leg Raises

- Starting Position:

Sit tall in the chair with feet flat on the floor.

- Steps:

Lift one leg to the side, keeping it straight, then lower it back down. Alternate legs.

- Repetition:

8-10 raises per leg.

- Purpose:

Targets the outer thigh muscles (abductors), improving hip strength and stability.

22. Seated Cat-Cow Stretch

- Starting Position:

Sit comfortably in the chair with hands resting on thighs.

- Steps:

Inhale, arch your back and lift your chest (Cow). Exhale, round your spine, tucking your chin towards your chest (Cat). Repeat the sequence.

- Repetition:

5-6 cycles.

- Purpose:

Increases spine mobility, stretches the back muscles, and promotes flexibility.

23. Seated Tricep Dips

- Starting Position:

Sit on the edge of the chair, place hands beside hips, gripping the edge of the seat.

- Steps:

Lift your body slightly off the chair, bending your elbows as you lower yourself down. Push back up to the starting position.

- Repetition:

8-10 tricep dips.

- Purpose:

Strengthens the triceps, improves arm strength, and enhances upper body stability.

24. Seated Hamstring Stretch

- Starting Position:

Sit on the chair's edge, one leg extended forward with the heel on the floor and the toes pointing upwards.

- Steps:

Lean forward from your hips, reaching towards your toes while keeping the back straight, feeling a stretch in the back of the extended leg.

- Repetition:

Hold the stretch for 20-30 seconds per leg, repeating 2-3 times.

- Purpose:

Stretches the hamstrings, improves leg flexibility, and eases tension in the lower body.

25. Seated Ankle Flex and Point

- Starting Position:

Sit tall with feet flat on the floor.

- Steps:

Flex your feet, pulling the toes towards your body, then point your toes away from you. Repeat the movement.

- Repetition:

Perform 10-12 flex and point movements.

- Purpose:

Increases ankle mobility, strengthens the lower leg muscles, and improves circulation in the feet and ankles.

26. Seated Side Leg Circles

- Starting Position:

Sit tall in the chair with feet flat on the floor.

- Steps:

Lift one leg slightly off the floor and make small circular motions with the extended leg. Reverse the direction after several circles. Alternate legs.

- Repetition:

6-8 circles in each direction per leg.

- Purpose:

Improves hip mobility, strengthens hip muscles, and enhances leg coordination.

27. Seated Arm Pulls

- Starting Position:

Sit comfortably with feet flat on the floor and arms extended forward at shoulder height.

- Steps:

Pull your elbows back, squeezing the shoulder blades together. Extend the arms back to the starting position.

- Repetition:

10-12 arm pulls.

- Purpose:

Strengthens the upper back muscles, improves posture, and counteracts slouching.

28. Seated Pelvic Clocks

- Starting Position:

Sit comfortably in the chair with feet flat on the floor.

- Steps:

Imagine the seat of the chair as the center of a clock. Move your hips in a circular motion as if tracing the numbers of the clock. Reverse the direction.

- Repetition:

4-6 circles in each direction.

- Purpose:

Enhances awareness of pelvic movement, promotes hip mobility, and improves core stability.

29. Seated Arm Crosses

- Starting Position:

Sit tall with feet flat on the floor and arms extended out to the sides at shoulder height.

- Steps:

Cross one arm over the other in front of your body, then return to the starting position. Alternate crossing arms.

- Repetition:

8-10 arm crosses per side.

- Purpose:

Engages the chest and shoulder muscles, improving shoulder flexibility and mobility.

30. Seated Full Body Stretch

- Starting Position:

Sit upright in the chair, feet flat on the floor, and hands resting on thighs.

- Steps:

Inhale deeply, reaching arms overhead, stretching upwards. Exhale as you lean slightly to one side, feeling a stretch along the torso. Return to center and repeat on the other side.

- Repetition:

Hold each side stretch for 15-20 seconds, repeating 2-3 times.

- Purpose:

Stretches the entire body, improves overall flexibility, and promotes relaxation.

CONCLUSION

Chair pilates for men over 50 is more than just a workout routine; it's a gateway to revitalizing both body and mind. Throughout this tailored exercise regimen, the focus remains on improving strength, flexibility, and mobility, all while seated comfortably. This holistic approach caters to the specific needs of men in this age group, providing a low-impact yet highly effective fitness solution.

The myriad of chair pilates exercises introduced here offers a comprehensive range of movements. From gentle stretches to targeted muscle engagement, each exercise aims to enhance physical well-being and address common issues faced by men over 50, such as joint stiffness, reduced flexibility, and posture concerns. Through consistent practice, individuals experience an improvement in core strength, increased flexibility, and better balance, leading to a more active and fulfilling lifestyle.

However, beyond the physical benefits, chair pilates offers an opportunity for mental rejuvenation. By focusing on controlled movements and mindful breathing, this practice cultivates a deeper mind-body connection. It fosters mental clarity, reduces stress, and promotes a sense of overall well-being, crucial for maintaining a positive outlook on life.

To all the men over 50 considering chair pilates, let this be your motivation: Embrace this journey not just as a means to improve physical fitness but as a path to rediscover your vitality and inner strength. Every stretch, every movement brings you closer to a more flexible, stronger, and healthier you. Remember, it's never too late to start investing in your well-being. Chair pilates offers a gentle, accessible, and highly rewarding way to reclaim your physical and mental vitality.

So, set aside any hesitation, start slowly, listen to your body, and embrace this transformative journey with determination. With commitment and dedication, chair pilates can become a cornerstone of your journey towards a more vibrant and fulfilling life, empowering you to age gracefully while enjoying improved health and vitality.

FITNESS

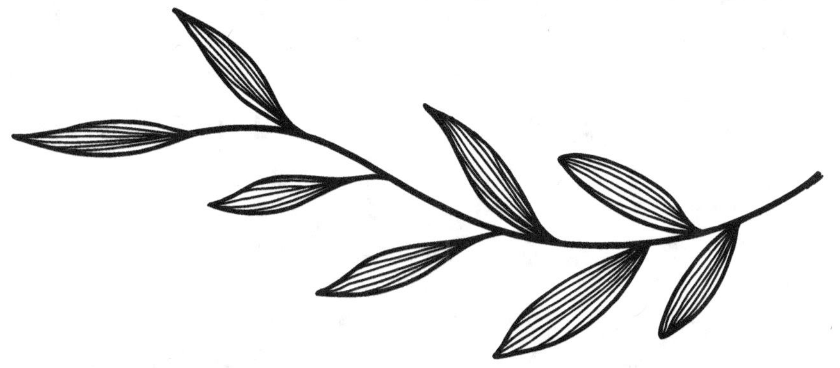

PLANNER

Fitness Planner

NAME: **DATE:**

BREAKFAST   ## LUNCH

DINNER   ## SNACK

EXERCISE   SET   REP   NOTES

Fitness Planner

NAME: **DATE:**

BREAKFAST

LUNCH

DINNER

SNACK

EXERCISE

EXERCISE	SET	REP	NOTES

Fitness Planner

NAME: **DATE:**

BREAKFAST   ### LUNCH

DINNER   ### SNACK

EXERCISE   SET   REP   NOTES

Fitness Planner

NAME: **DATE:**

BREAKFAST

LUNCH

DINNER

SNACK

EXERCISE

SET

REP

NOTES

Fitness Planner

NAME: DATE:

BREAKFAST

LUNCH

DINNER

SNACK

EXERCISE	SET	REP	NOTES

Fitness Planner

NAME: **DATE:**

BREAKFAST

LUNCH

DINNER

SNACK

EXERCISE

SET	REP	NOTES

Fitness Planner

NAME: **DATE:**

BREAKFAST

LUNCH

DINNER

SNACK

EXERCISE   SET   REP   NOTES

Fitness Planner

NAME:

DATE:

BREAKFAST

LUNCH

DINNER

SNACK

EXERCISE

SET

REP

NOTES

Fitness Planner

NAME: **DATE:**

BREAKFAST

LUNCH

DINNER

SNACK

EXERCISE | SET | REP | NOTES

Fitness Planner

NAME:

DATE:

BREAKFAST

LUNCH

DINNER

SNACK

EXERCISE

SET

REP

NOTES

www.ingramcontent.com/pod-product-compliance
Lightning Source LLC
Chambersburg PA
CBHW071105260726
48661CB00006B/2477